Beary the Anxious Bear

by Mohammed Ahmed

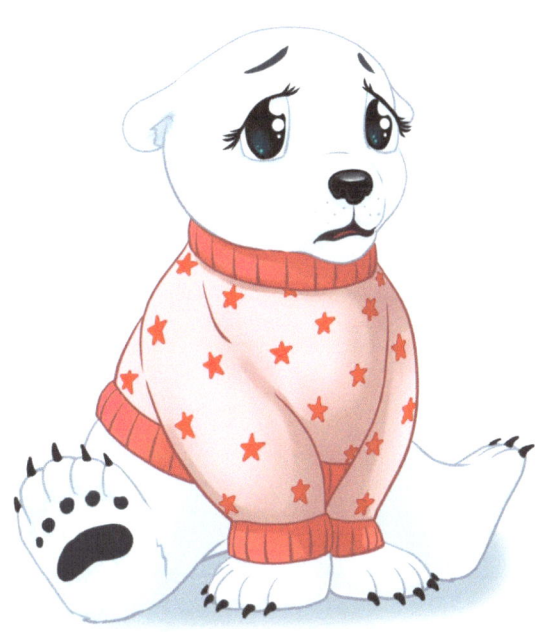

Illustrated by Irena Urosevic

There are times when things happen to us that make us develop anxiety. It may be an upcoming dance or a basketball game in school. It may even be that we are lost in the store and need to find mom and dad.

Anxiety is a feeling that we have when we feel that something bad has happened or will happen. It is the way we feel when we think that what has not happened would happen.

Let me tell you the story of Beary the anxious bear and how her friend, Victoria, helped her deal with the anxiety.

Once upon a time there was a bear called Beary. Beary was a beautiful bear with white fur and beautiful eyes. She was four years old.

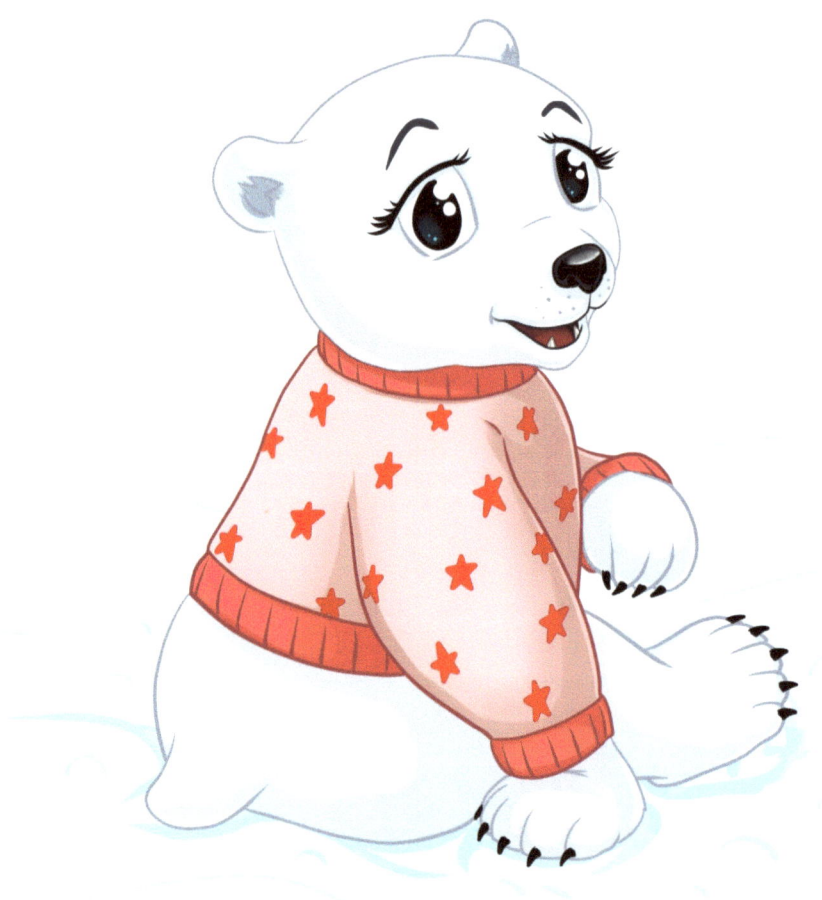

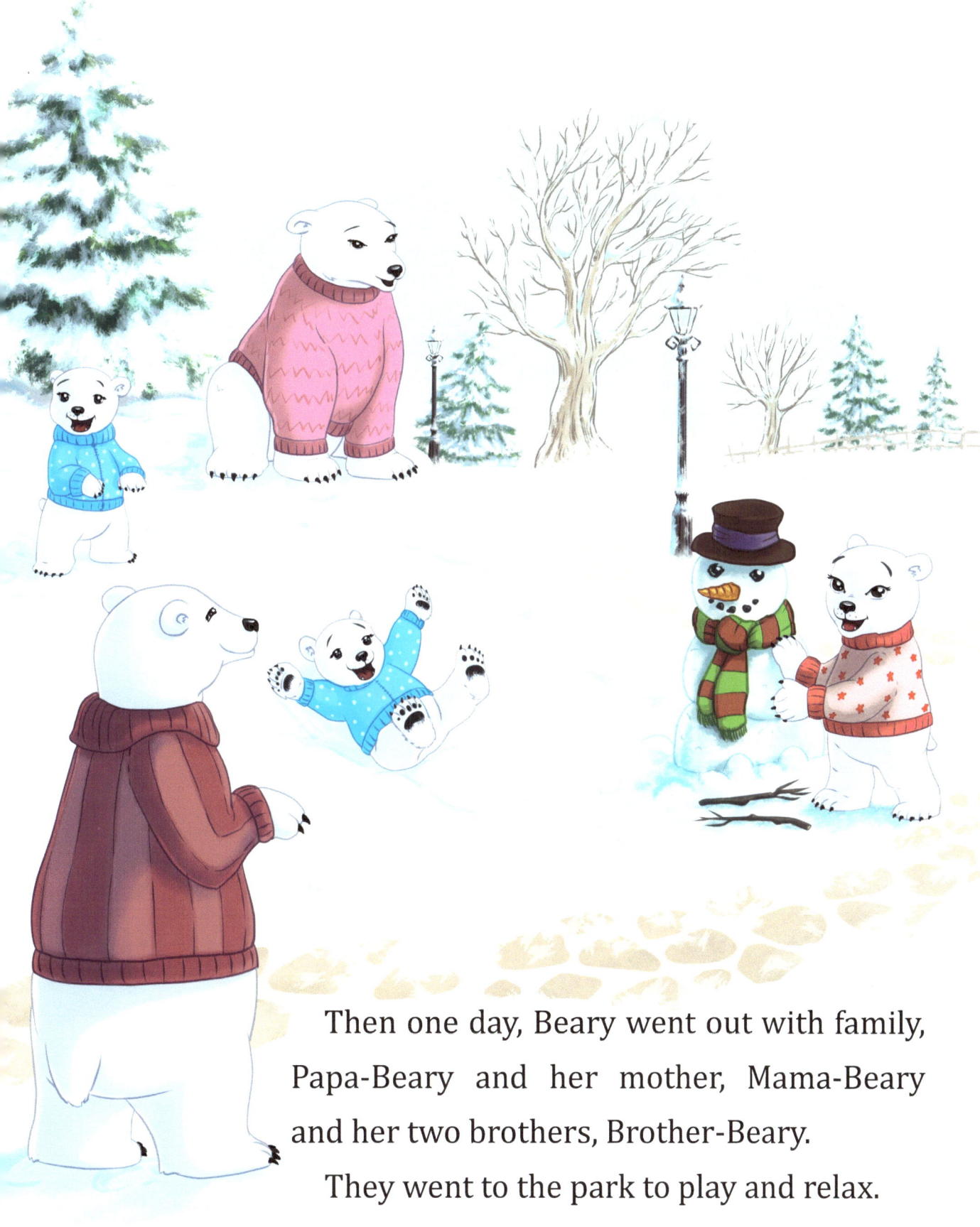

Then one day, Beary went out with family, Papa-Beary and her mother, Mama-Beary and her two brothers, Brother-Beary.

They went to the park to play and relax.

When they got to the park, the young Beary left her family to go play in the woods alone.

She wandered into the thick part of the Woods. After she returned to the park, she could not find her mother and father and brothers again. She became very worried. She was scared and very anxious that she would not see her parents again.

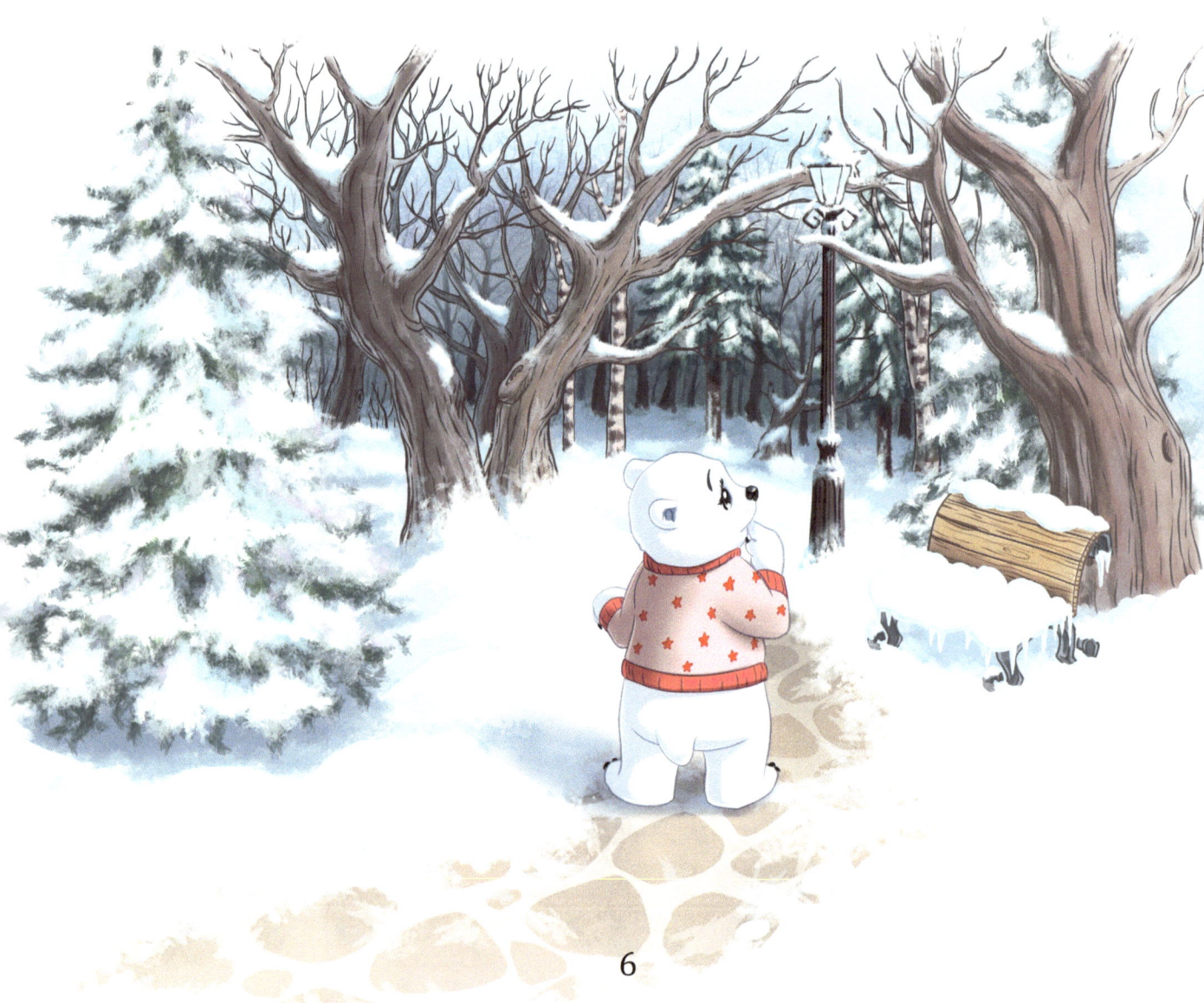

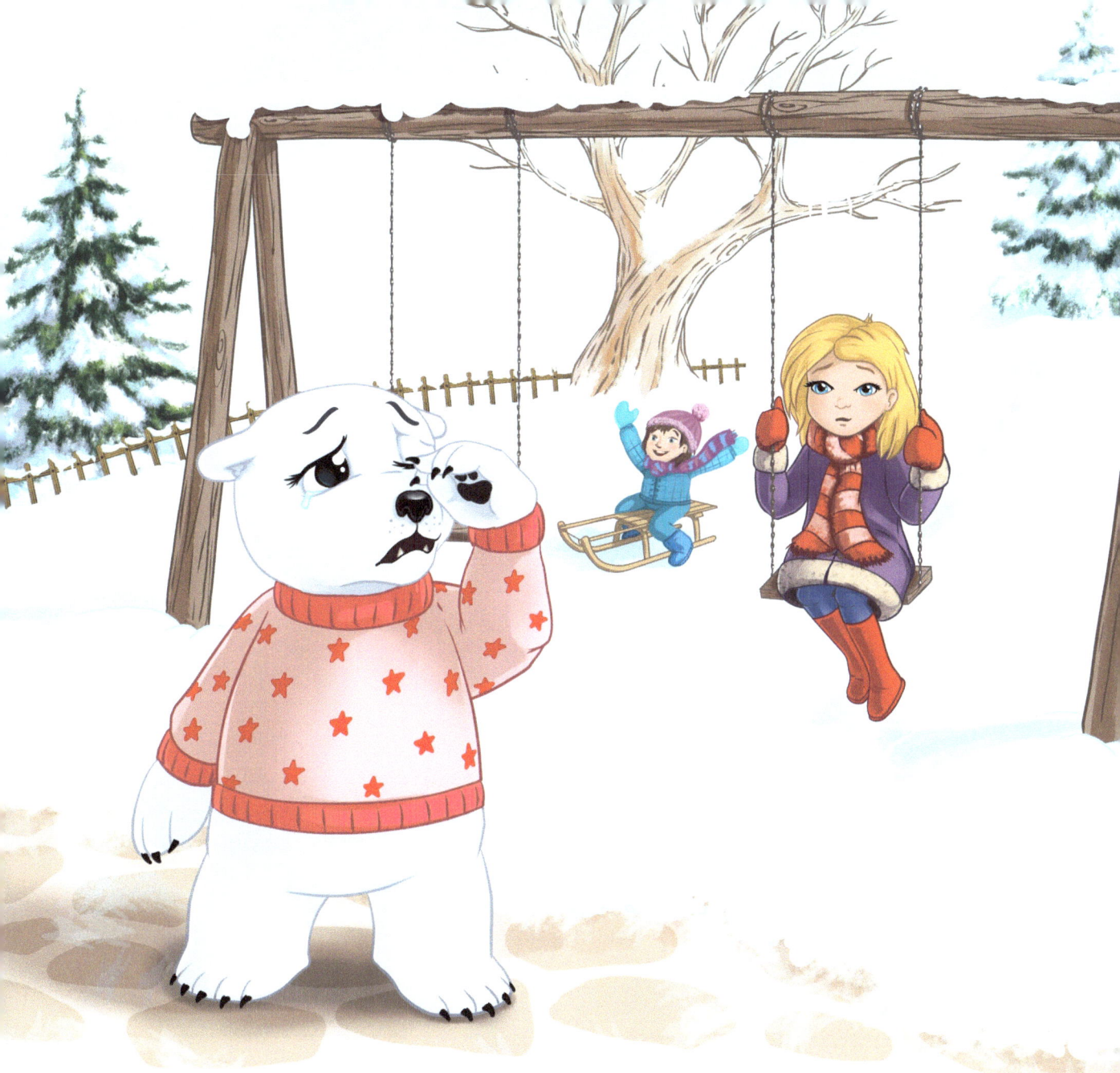

Beary was confused. She did not know what to do. She was about to start crying when she saw a very beautiful girl who had beautiful red boots. The girl saw Beary anxious and close to tears, and she walked up to Beary with a smile on her face.

Girl: Hi, my name is Victoria, what's your name?

Beary: My name is Beary, I cannot find my parents.

Victoria: Oh, that's sad, Beary.

Beary: And I'm getting very worried.

Victoria: I know how you feel. I will help you find them.

Beary: You will? Oh, thank you.

Victoria: No problem Beary. I'll be your friend and help you find your parents and brothers.

Beary: So where do we start, I'm anxious right now.

Victoria: I Know Beary, everybody gets anxious.

Beary: So what do I do? I need to find them.

Victoria: First, would you allow me help you stop being anxious? We can't do much if you're anxious.

Beary: Really, we can't?

Victoria: Yes dear Beary, we can't.

Beary: Why is that?

Victoria: Because when you are anxious you would not be able to think properly. Your mind would be very confused.

Beary: Really?

Victoria: Yes. So you have to let me help you stop being anxious.

Beary: Okay, Victoria.

Victoria: Beary, what happened to your parents and brothers, how are they missing?

Beary tells Victoria about how she left them in the park and wandered into the woods alone. She did not know how long she spent in the woods, but when she came back she could not find them anymore.

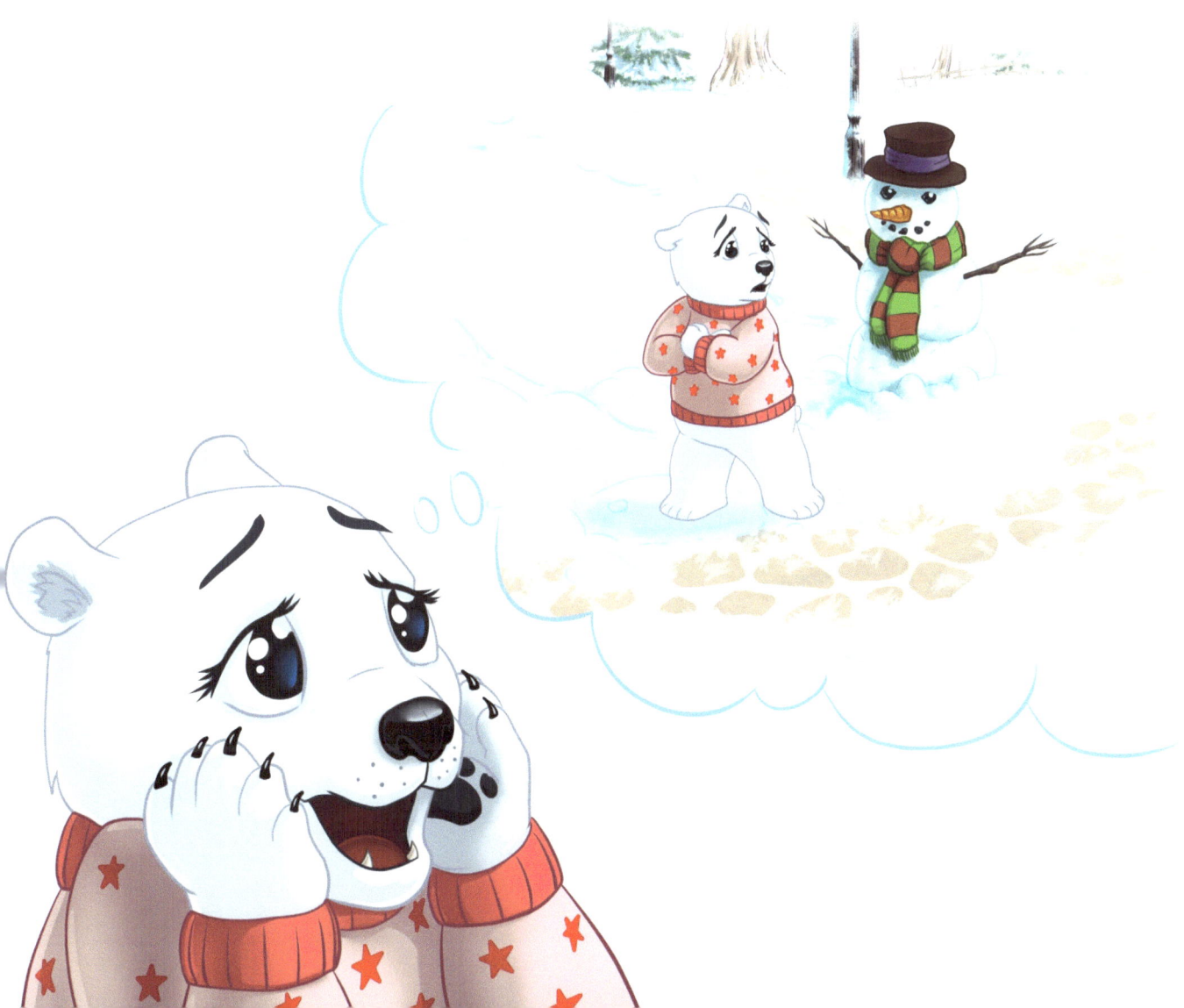

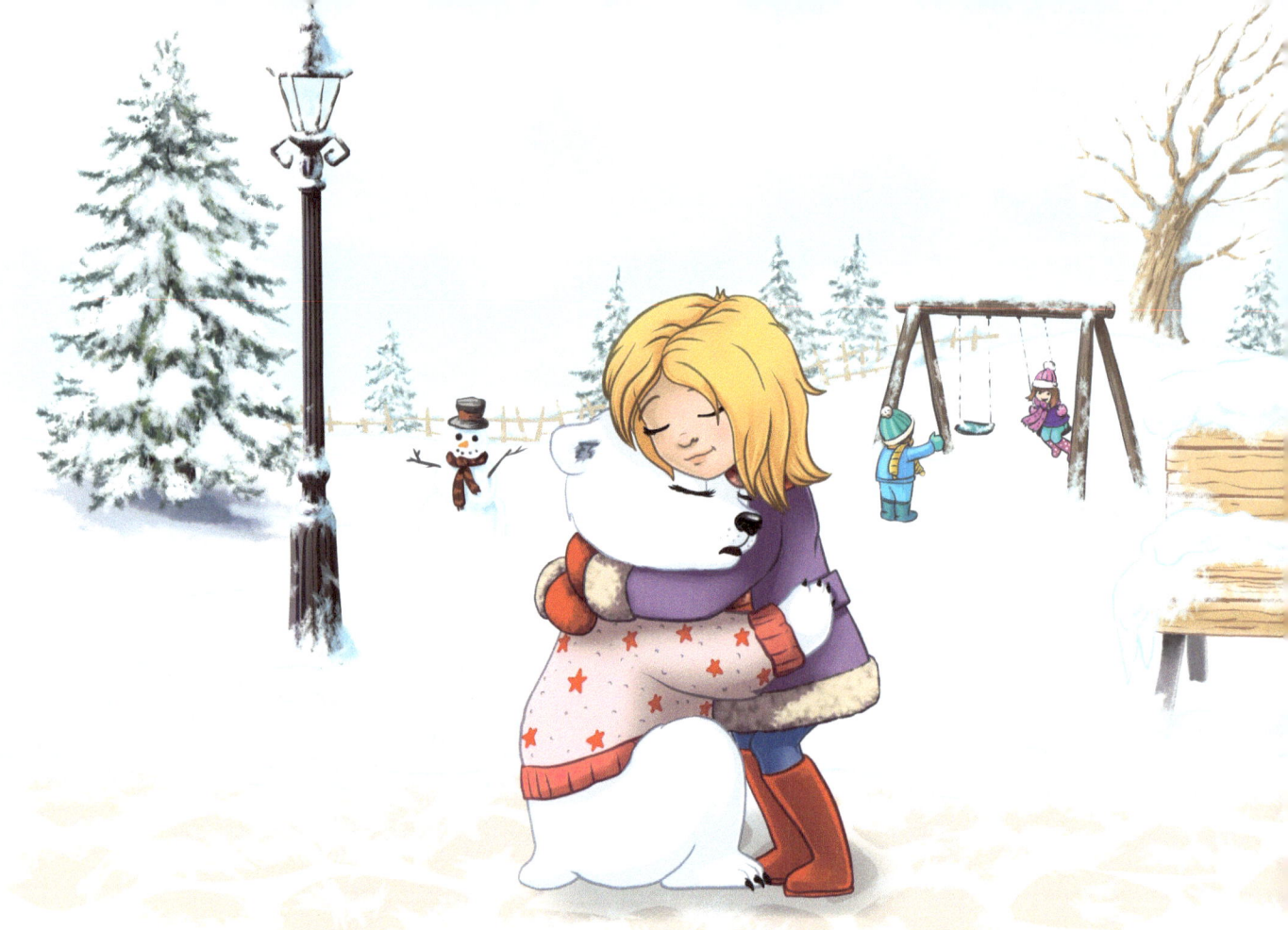

Victoria listened to her attentively and when Beary finished explaining, Victoria looked at her and hugged Beary.

Victoria: Do you think they too have gone missing?

Beary: I don't know.

Victoria: What if they are now looking for you, since you didn't tell them where it was you were going.

Beary: Yeaah. That is true. My Mama and Papa might be looking for me too.

Victoria: You see, they haven't been stolen. They are fine.

Beary: You are right Victoria, thank you. I feel better now after talking to you.

Victoria took Beary to the swings and played while Beary waited for her parents and brothers to come back.

They had played for a while but Beary's parents did not come.

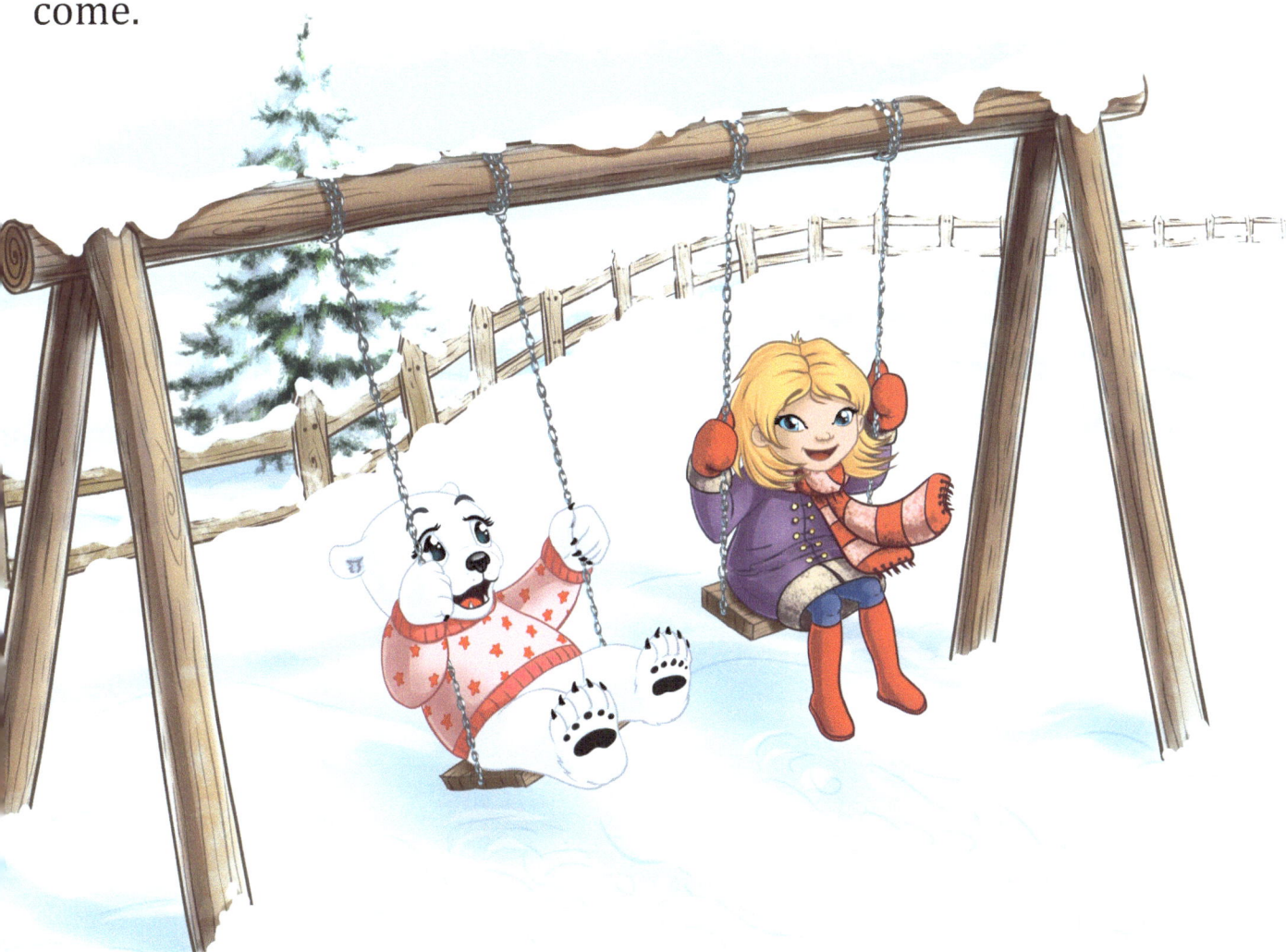

Beary: Victoria, they haven't come, what should I do?

Victoria: Hmm. Are you anxious again?

Beary: Yes I am. It is almost getting dark and they've not come back here. Where could they be?

Victoria: Maybe they are still looking for you. Let's see if we can find them ourselves.

Beary: Thank you Victoria, you are a real friend.

Victoria: No problem Beary, we will find them. I just need you to be relaxed.

Beary: I am already.

Victoria: No you're not. You're anxious. I am going to teach you the breathing technique to help you stop being anxious, are you ready?

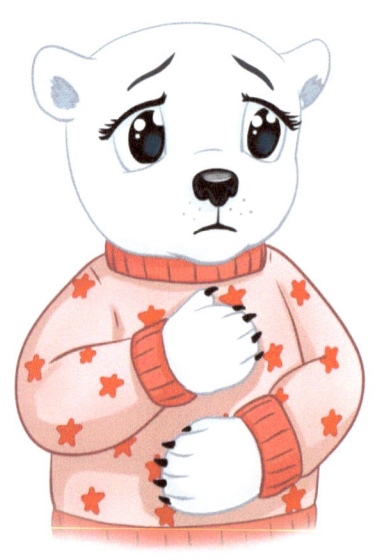

Beary: Ready like Beary.

Victoria: Haha, that's good Beary. Let's try this together.

Beary: Okay Victoria.

Victoria: Place one of your hands on your chest, and another one below your waistline, close to your stomach.

Beary did as she was instructed.

Victoria: Good. Do you know why I told you to place your hands there?

Beary: No, I don't.

Victoria: I want you to notice how your breathing changes when you breathe in deep. Your breathing affects how much anxiety you feel.

Beary: That's good.

Victoria: Open your mouth, and sigh. Sigh like somebody just told you, you couldn't have candy anymore and want to pull off your fur.

Beary sighed.

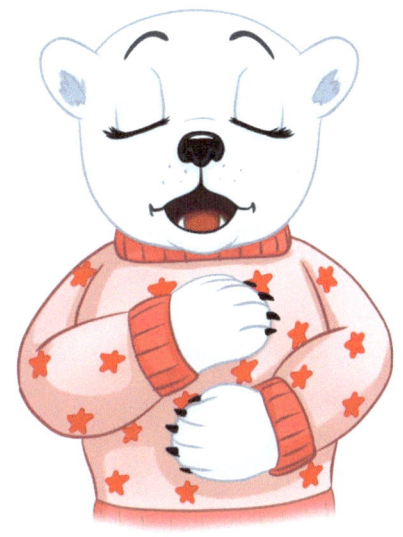

Victoria: Good. I like that. Now, let your shoulders down. Let them come down like you just found that candy you've been looking for.

Beary let her shoulders fall.

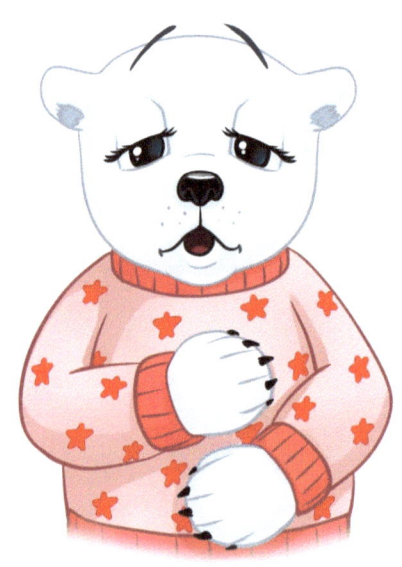

Victoria: Now close your mouth.

Beary: Okay.

Victoria: You're not supposed to be talking Beary.

Beary: Hmmmmm.

Victoria: Hmmmmm. Good.

Beary smiled.

Victoria: Take a deep breath through your nose, like this.

Beary: Like this?

Victoria: No, no. Not like that. Push your stomach forward a bit and use your nose to drag in all the air in the room: Like this.

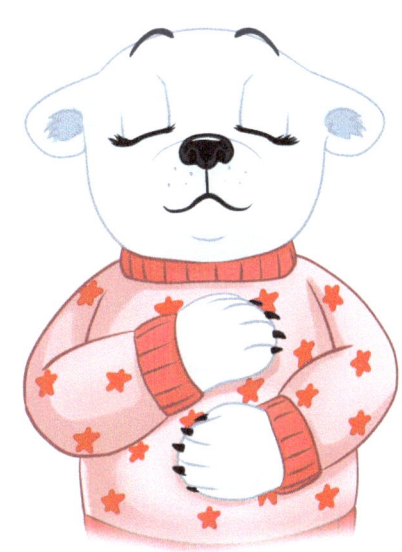

Beary took a deep breath. Victoria smiles at her, she gets it right.

Victoria: Don't let go. Hold on to that air you've inhaled. Just a little longer. Two more seconds. Good.

Beary did as she said.

Victoria: Open your mouth now, slowly and breathe out through your mouth.

Beary: Haaaaaa.

Victoria: Very good Beary, you did it right. How do you feel now?

Beary: I feel... I feel... More relaxed than before. Thank you Victoria.

Victoria: No problem, that's what friends are for.

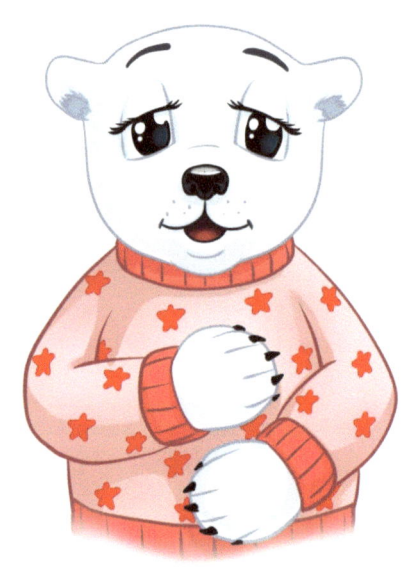

After that, they left the park in search of Beary's parents. After they had walked a few miles with no sign of her parents, Beary began to sweat. Victoria looked at her with a lot of concern in her eyes.

She is such a good friend.

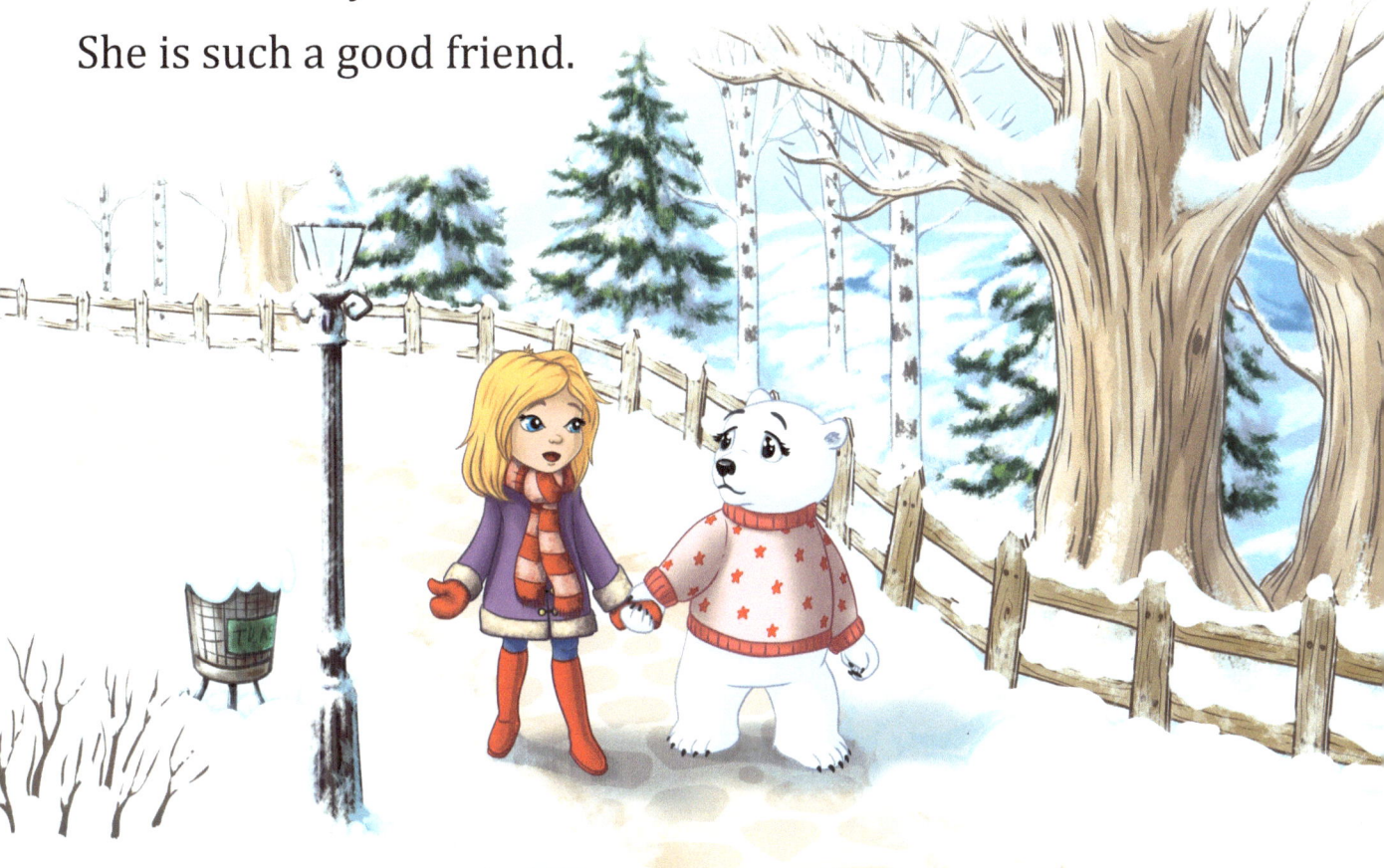

Victoria: Beary, what do you fear would happen to your family?

Beary: I don't know, maybe...

Victoria: I'm your friend Beary, you can tell me what you fear would be the worst thing that could happen to your family.

Beary: I fear they might go missing for life.

Victoria: For life? Why would you think so?

Beary: I heard that the forest is dangerous at night.

Victoria: Who told you that?

Beary: A friend of mine. He said people get lost in the forest a lot.

Victoria: That's not true Beary. There are guards in the forest who protect the area. They won't allow anything bad happen to your family.

Beary: Are you sure?

Victoria: I am sure. Just be calm.

Beary: Okay, I will.

Victoria: Let's do another breathing exercise to help you get calm. I have a feeling we will see your family very soon. You don't want to meet them while you're anxious, do you?

Beary: No, I don't.

Victoria: Let us sit down over there.

Beary: What kind of breathing are we doing this time? I liked the first one, it helped me relax.

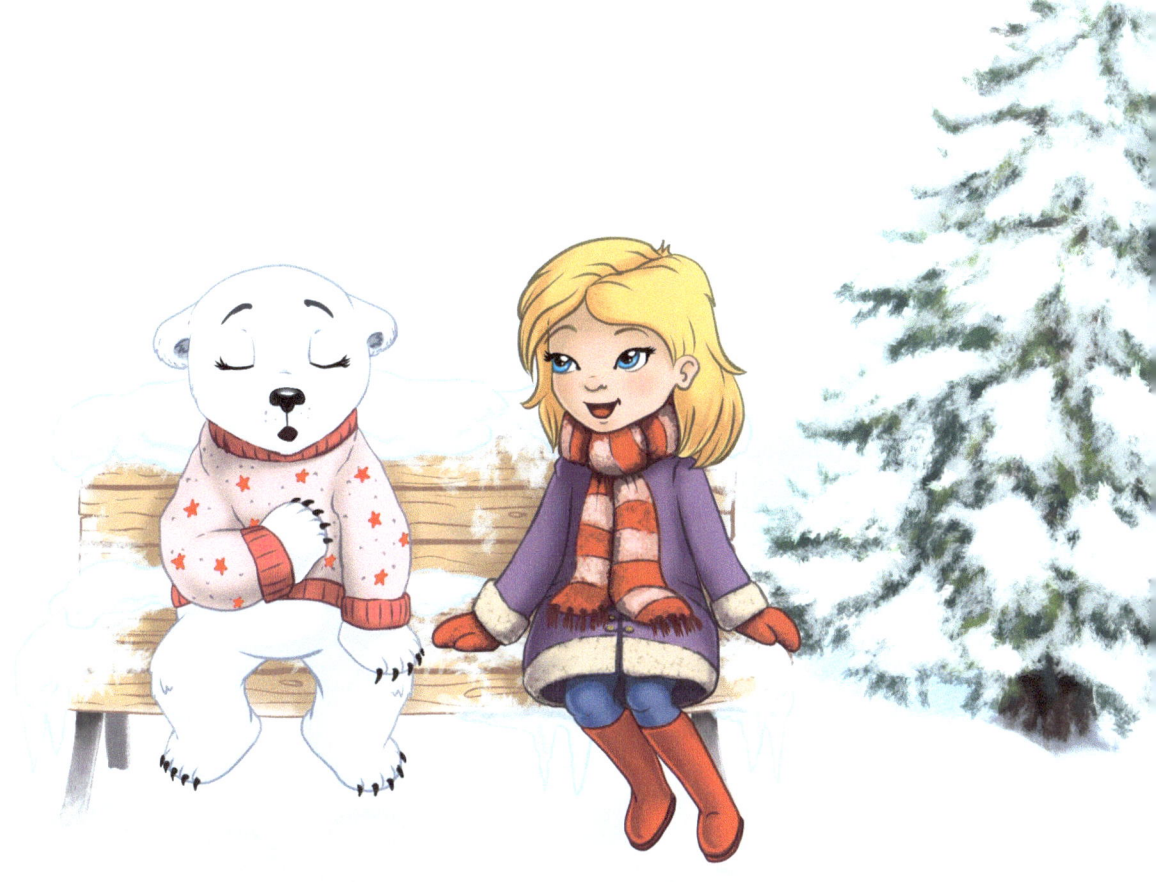

Victoria: Since we are seated, I want you to close your eyes.

Beary did as she was told. She really wants to be calm when she sees her parents and her brothers. She doesn't want them to think she can't take care of herself.

Victoria: That is very good. Now take a long deep breath. Do it like you would normally breathe. Open your mouth slightly to take in enough air.

Victoria: That's good Beary. You are doing it right. I want you to breathe out slowly, and say softly "relax Beary".

Beary exhaled slowly saying "relax Beary".

She smiled after the first round of deep breathing and exhaling.

Victoria: Keep doing it. Do it ten more times: Inhale, and exhale.

Beary sat there with her eyes shut and kept inhaling and exhaling, while she said, "relax Beary". When Victoria saw that it was more than ten times, she tapped Beary softly on her shoulder.

Victoria: It has passed the ten times I told you to.

Beary: Oh it has? I was enjoying it. It made feel very calm now. I am ready to find my parents and brothers now. I'm sure I'll find them.

Victoria: That's good Beary. You see, it is not as bad as you thought. We will find your parents and your brothers.

Victoria: Everything will be okay!

While they stood up to leave, Beary saw a man with a guard uniform walking towards them.

Beary: Victoria, a guard. A guard is coming towards us. What do we do?

Victoria: Let's ask him if he has seen your parents and your brothers.

They waited for the guard to come to them.

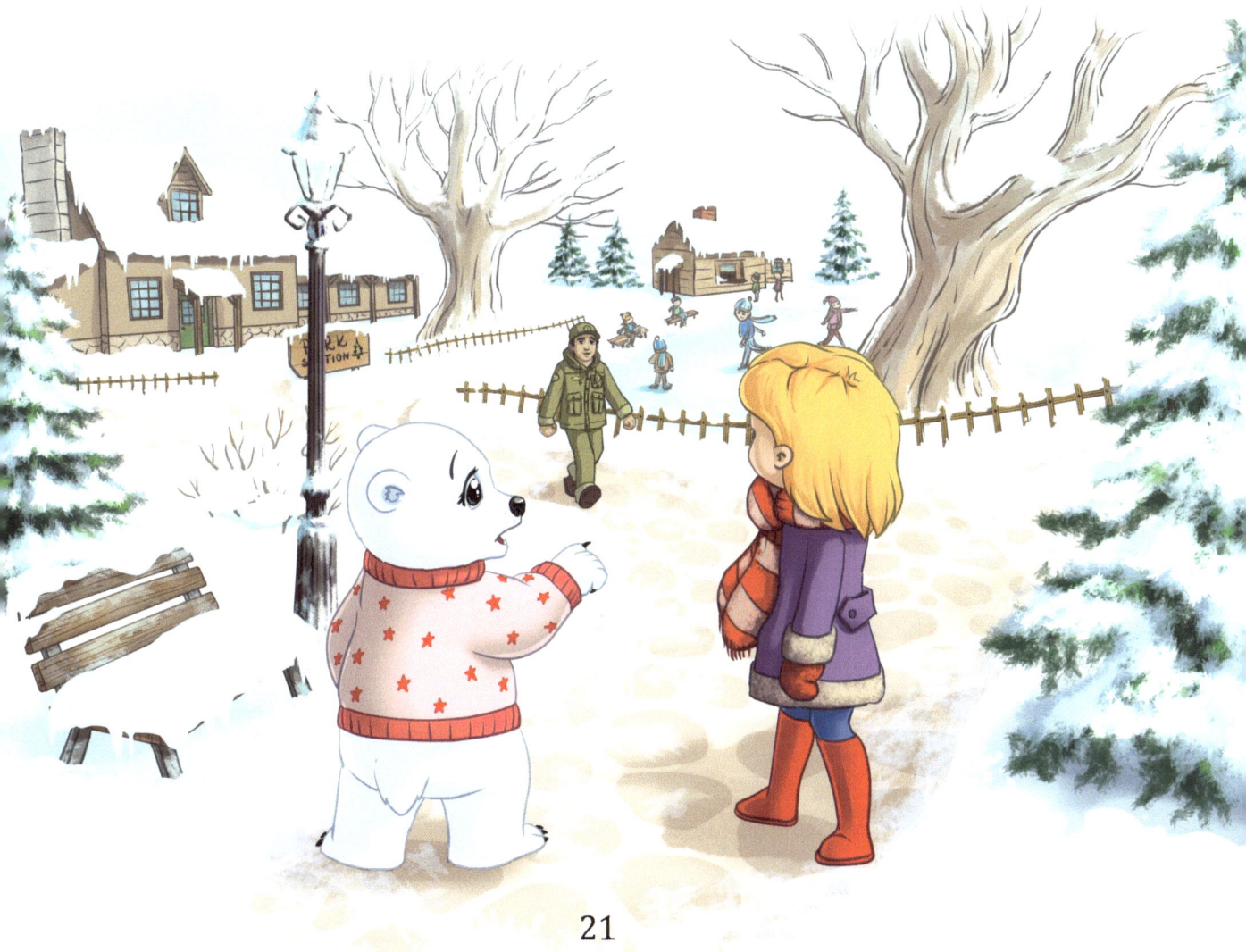

Guard: What are you two doing here? It is almost dark and you should not be here.

Beary: Sir, I left my parents and brothers at the park and wandered into the woods. I did not tell them where I was going. When I returned to the park, I did not see them again. I've been looking for them.

Victoria: Please sir, have you seen them around? I suspect they are also looking for Beary.

The guard told them he had seen Beary's parents and brothers. They were at the park station. He took Beary and Victoria to see her family.

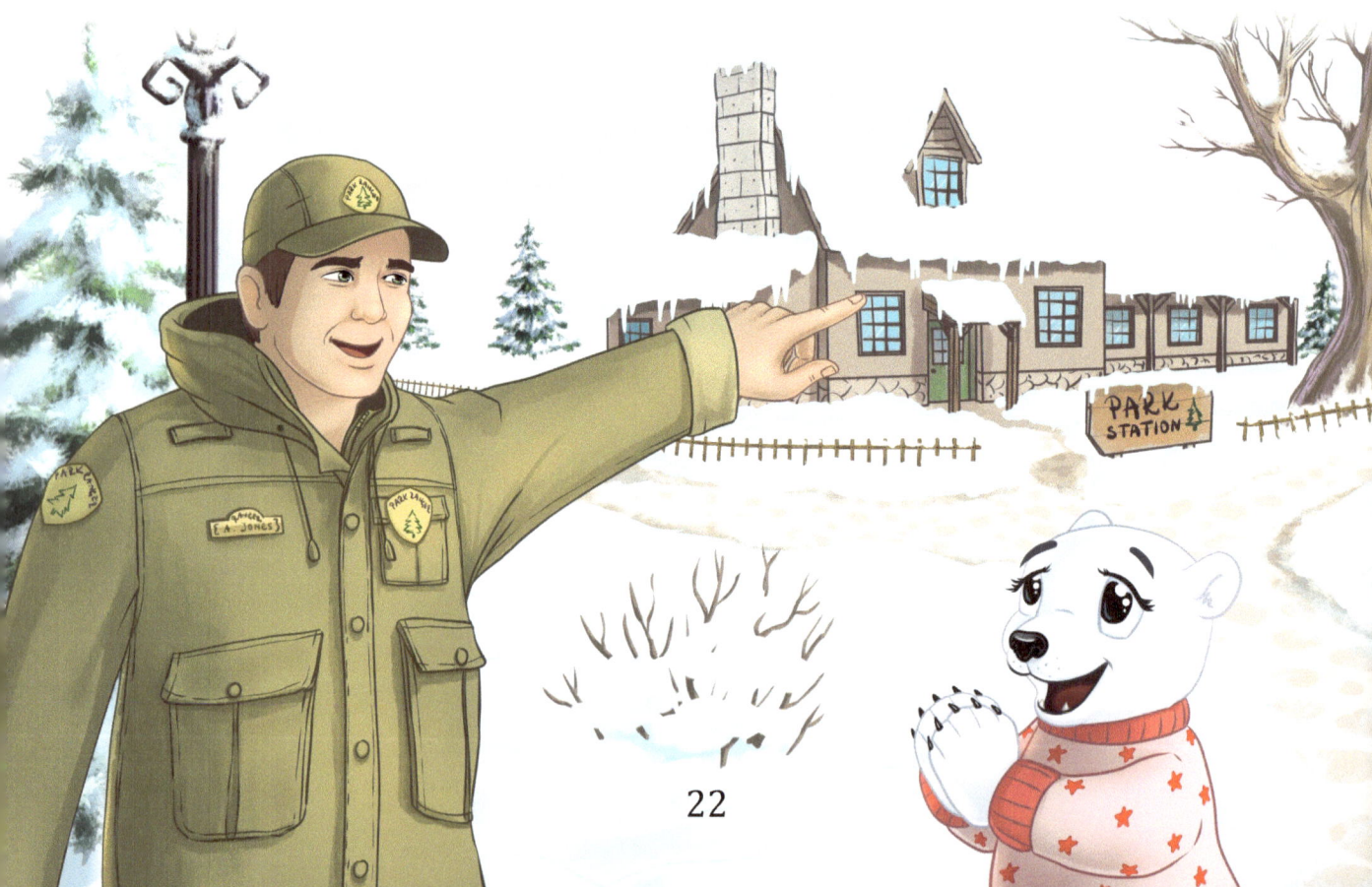

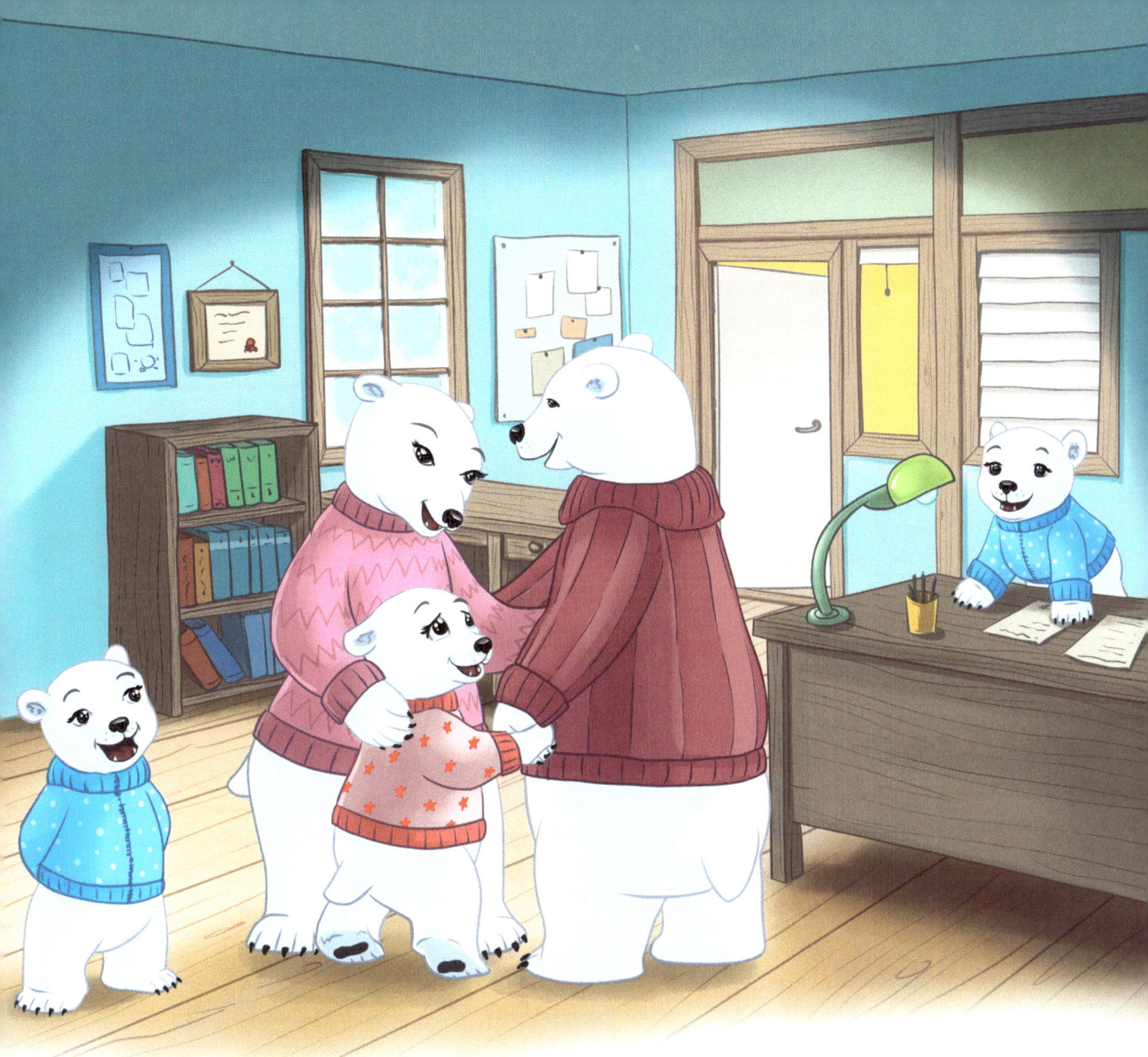

Beary was very happy when she saw her parents and her two brothers. She apologized to them. She also told them about her new friend, Victoria, who helped her deal with her anxiety. Beary's parents were very happy and thanked Victoria for helping Beary keep calm when she was anxious.

When they wanted to leave, Beary rushed to hug Victoria again and then Victoria looked at her.

Victoria: Beary, I want you to always remember the breathing exercise I taught you. Whenever you feel anxious, take a deep breathe and then remember you have a friend who loves you. Okay?

Beary: Okay. Thank you Victoria!

Victoria: Until next time Beary...

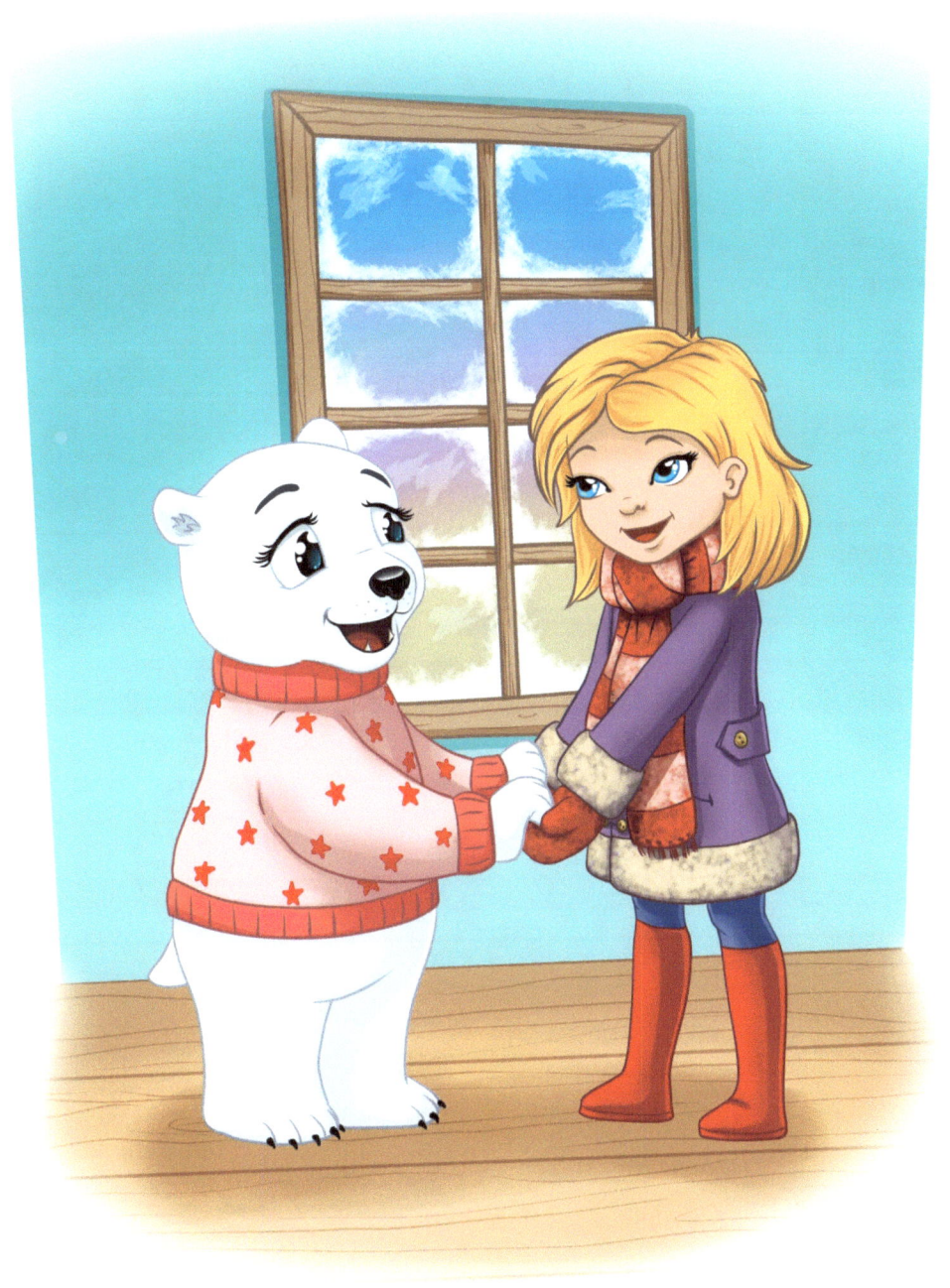

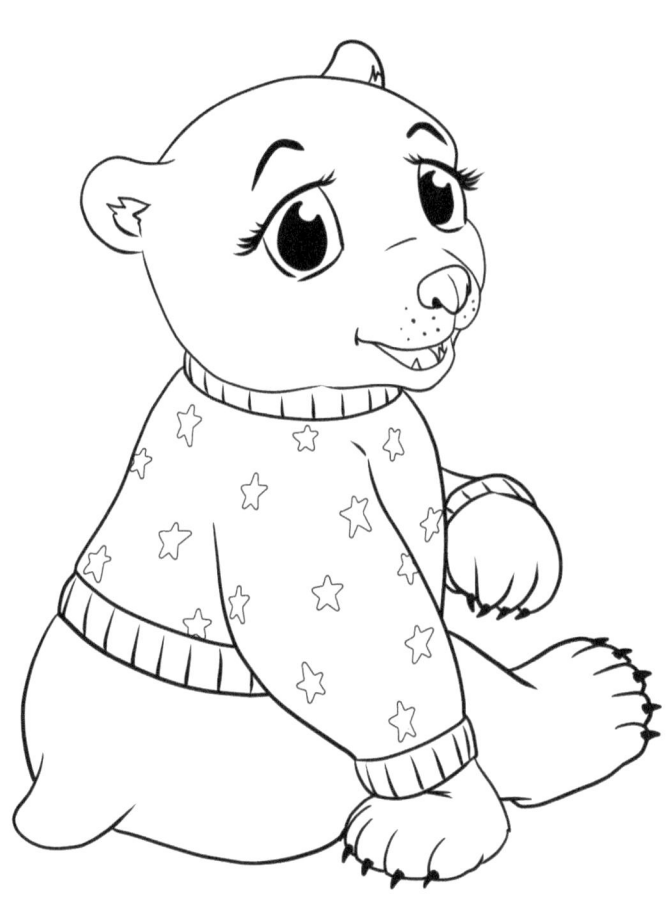

www.ingramcontent.com/pod-product-compliance
Lightning Source LLC
Chambersburg PA
CBHW060818290526
45792CB00005BB/1714